BE YOUR OWN DOCTOR: A GUIDE TO

SELF-CARE AND WELLNESS

I0446728

The Ultimate Guide to Self-Care, Wellness

Mastery, and Taking Control of your

Health

Dorothy L. Richey

CONTENTS

CONTENTS   2

INTRODUCTION   7

THE POWER OF BEING YOUR OWN DOCTOR   7

CHAPTER ONE   13

UNDERSTANDING YOUR BODY – THE MIRACULOUS MACHINE WITHIN   13
THE HUMAN BODY: A MARVEL OF ENGINEERING   13
A TOUR THROUGH THE BODY   14
THE SYMPHONY OF LIFE   17
WHY UNDERSTANDING YOUR BODY MATTERS?   18

CHAPTER TWO   21

NOURISHING YOUR WAY TO WELLNESS: THE ART OF NUTRITION AND DIET   21
CREATING A BALANCED DIET   22
SPECIAL DIETS FOR SPECIFIC NEEDS   27

CHAPTER THREE   35

UNLOCKING YOUR POTENTIAL: THE TRANSFORMATIVE POWER OF EXERCISE AND
PHYSICAL ACTIVITY   35
THE BENEFITS OF EXERCISE   35
CREATING AN EXERCISE ROUTINE   37
STAYING ACTIVE THROUGHOUT LIFE   38

CHAPTER FOUR   41

HARMONY WITHIN: NURTURING MENTAL HEALTH AND STRESS MANAGEMENT FOR
A BALANCED LIFE   41
MIND-BODY CONNECTION   41
COPING WITH STRESS   45
STRATEGIES FOR MAINTAINING GOOD MENTAL HEALTH   48

CHAPTER FIVE   51

INVEST IN YOUR HEALTH: THE POWER OF PREVENTIVE CARE   51
THE IMPORTANCE OF PREVENTIVE HEALTH MEASURES   51
REGULAR CHECK-UPS AND SCREENINGS   52
VACCINATIONS AND IMMUNIZATIONS   53
THE ECONOMICS OF PREVENTIVE CARE   55

CHAPTER SIX   57

COMMON AILMENTS AND HOME REMEDIES: YOUR ULTIMATE GUIDE TO SELF-CARE
      57
SELF-CARE FOR MINOR ILLNESSES   58
IN ALL CASES: 61
FIRST AID TECHNIQUES   62
HERBAL REMEDIES AND ALTERNATIVE THERAPIES   67
EMPOWER YOURSELF WITH KNOWLEDGE   68

CHAPTER SEVEN   69

CHRONIC DISEASE MANAGEMENT: TAKING CONTROL OF YOUR HEALTH   69
MEDICATION MANAGEMENT: YOUR PILLARS OF SUPPORT   70
LIFESTYLE CHANGES FOR CHRONIC CONDITIONS: YOUR PATH TO A BRIGHTER
TOMORROW   71

CHAPTER EIGHT   75

EMPOWERING YOURSELF THROUGH SELF-DIAGNOSIS AND SYMPTOM
MANAGEMENT   75
IDENTIFYING SYMPTOMS   76
ONLINE HEALTH RESOURCES   80
WHEN TO SEEK PROFESSIONAL HELP   85

CHAPTER NINE   91

THE HEALING POWER OF NATURE: HERBAL MEDICINE AND ALTERNATIVE THERAPIES
                                                                    91
HERBAL REMEDIES: THE GIFTS OF THE EARTH   91
ACUPUNCTURE AND AYURVEDA: ANCIENT WISDOM IN MODERN TIMES   92
INTEGRATING ALTERNATIVE AND CONVENTIONAL MEDICINE: A NEW PARADIGM   93
A BALANCING ACT: CHOOSING THE RIGHT PATH   95

CHAPTER TEN   97

BUILDING A HOLISTIC HEALTH PLAN: A PATH TO WELLNESS AND VITALITY   97
PERSONALIZED HEALTH GOALS: CRAFTING YOUR WELLNESS BLUEPRINT   97
DEVELOPING A WELLNESS ROUTINE: NURTURING YOUR MIND AND BODY   99
STAYING INFORMED AND ADAPTING: THE DYNAMIC NATURE OF HEALTH   101

CHAPTER ELEVEN   103

MEDICAL EMERGENCIES AND WHEN TO SEEK PROFESSIONAL HELP.   103
RECOGNIZING TRUE EMERGENCIES   103
WHEN TO CALL 911   105
PREPARING FOR MEDICAL APPOINTMENTS   106

CHAPTER TWELVE   109

THE FUTURE OF SELF-CARE AND HEALTH TECH   109
TELEMEDICINE AND HEALTH APPS   109
THE ROLE OF AI IN HEALTHCARE   111
THE EVOLVING LANDSCAPE OF SELF-CARE   112

CONCLUSION   115

EMPOWERING YOURSELF AS A HEALTH ADVOCATE   115
STRIKING A BALANCE BETWEEN SELF-CARE AND PROFESSIONAL CARE 116

INTRODUCTION

The Power of Being Your Own Doctor

In the grand tapestry of life, our health is the most precious thread. It's the one thing we often take for granted until, like a fragile silk strand, it begins to unravel. Suddenly, we are confronted with the daunting reality of illness or discomfort, a harsh reminder of the fragility of existence. But what if I told you that within the very fabric of your being, you possess the power to mend those unravelling threads? What if you could take charge of your health, understand your body, and become your own doctor?

Welcome to "Be Your Own Doctor: A Guide to Self-Care and Wellness." This book is your compass through the labyrinth of well-being, designed to empower you with knowledge, inspire you to make informed choices, and guide you on a transformative journey of self-discovery and health optimization.

The concept of being your own doctor might sound unconventional in a world where we've been conditioned to rely on healthcare professionals for every ailment and discomfort. Don't get me wrong; doctors and medical practitioners play an invaluable role in our lives, and their expertise is irreplaceable. However, the idea that you can actively participate in your health and well-being is not about replacing medical expertise but rather about complementing it. It's about harnessing the innate wisdom of your body and mind to lead a healthier, happier life.

In these pages, you'll embark on an enlightening voyage of self-discovery. You'll learn about the remarkable complexity of your body, the interplay of its various systems, and the secrets to nourishing it properly. You'll uncover the profound connection between your mental and physical health, discover the art of stress management, and delve into the depths of preventive care.

This journey isn't just about the absence of disease; it's about the presence of vitality. It's about embracing wellness as a lifestyle, making conscious choices, and understanding that self-care is the foundation of a fulfilling existence.

It's often said that knowledge is power, and in the realm of healthcare, this adage couldn't be truer. When you understand how your body functions, how it responds to the foods you eat, the exercise you do, and the lifestyle you lead, you gain the power to influence your well-being positively. Imagine possessing the ability to prevent illness, manage minor health concerns, and make well-informed decisions about your health.

The 19th-century poet and philosopher, Ralph Waldo Emerson, once said, "The first wealth is health." Your health is the cornerstone of your life's journey, and by exploring the depths of self-care and wellness, you are not only investing in your health but also in the quality of your life, relationships, and dreams. This book equips you with the tools you need to begin building this wealth of health.

Wellness is more than just the absence of disease; it's the harmonious integration of physical, mental, and emotional well-being. In this book, we'll delve into a holistic approach to health and self-care, recognizing that every aspect of your life is interconnected. What you eat affects how you feel, how you manage stress impacts your physical health, and your mindset can influence your recovery.

By addressing health from a holistic perspective, we'll explore the profound interplay between body, mind, and spirit. You'll learn how to strike a balance that resonates with your unique being, optimizing your health on every level.

One of the most beautiful aspects of being your own doctor is the personalization of your health journey. There's no one-size-fits-all solution when it comes to well-being. Your body, your life, and your health are uniquely yours. This book empowers you to take charge of your health and tailor it to your specific needs.

We'll discuss the importance of personalized health goals and how to create a wellness routine that aligns with your aspirations. It's about building a health plan that isn't imposed upon you but one that you craft and refine over time, ensuring it resonates with who you are and what you desire.

The world of healthcare is constantly evolving, with advancements in medicine, technology, and research reshaping our understanding of the human body. In this book, we'll explore the future of self-care and how emerging trends such as telemedicine and health tech are revolutionizing the way we approach well-being.

We'll also discuss the vital role of artificial intelligence in healthcare, how it's enhancing diagnostics and treatment recommendations, and how you can harness this cutting-edge technology to be even more effective in being your own doctor.

Ultimately, the goal of this book is to empower you as a health advocate, to inspire you to take charge of your well-being with confidence and knowledge. It's about recognizing that you have the capacity to be your own doctor, not in the sense of having a medical degree but in the sense of being your primary caretaker, the guardian of your health.

The journey ahead is filled with insights, practical advice, and the wisdom of self-care. You'll learn about nutrition, exercise, mental health, preventive care, symptom management, and much more. Each chapter is a stepping stone on the path to greater wellness.

As you embark on this enlightening journey, I encourage you to approach it with an open mind and a willingness to explore new horizons. Your body is a remarkable, resilient vessel, and your mind is a powerful instrument. Together, they hold the keys to a healthier, happier, and more vibrant life.

So, are you ready to take that first step toward becoming your own doctor? Let's embark on this transformative journey of self-care and wellness together, as we unlock the incredible potential within you. Your well-being is worth the investment, and the rewards are boundless.

CHAPTER ONE

Understanding Your Body – The Miraculous Machine Within

Have you ever paused to marvel at the incredible complexity and perfection of the human body? Each day, it performs countless intricate processes, keeping you alive and functioning at your best. In this chapter, we'll take an exciting journey through the awe-inspiring world of human anatomy and physiology, helping you unlock the secrets of your body.

The Human Body: A Marvel of Engineering

Imagine for a moment that you are the proud owner of a state-of-the-art machine, one that's been meticulously designed over millions of years. This machine can heal itself, adapt to its environment, and even experience emotions and sensations. This machine is your body.

Your body is a masterpiece of engineering, a work of art sculpted by evolution itself. The moment you open your eyes in the morning, it springs into action, seamlessly coordinating billions of cells, muscles, and organs to perform tasks as varied as breathing, digestion, and thought. It's like a well-choreographed symphony, where every instrument plays its part to create the beautiful melody that is your life.

A Tour Through the Body

Let's embark on a guided tour of this magnificent creation.

Skeletal System: First stop, the framework of your body, the skeleton. It's not just a scaffold; it's a dynamic structure that produces blood cells and protects vital organs. With 206 bones in the adult human body, it provides support and allows you to move with grace and agility.

Muscular System: Next, we delve into the muscular system. Picture your muscles as the powerhouse of the body, converting energy into motion. From lifting a cup of coffee to running a marathon, it's your muscles that make it all possible.

Circulatory System: Now, let's explore the circulatory system. Imagine a network of rivers and streams crisscrossing your body, carrying vital nutrients and oxygen to every cell. This is your blood's journey, and your heart is the master pump that keeps it all flowing.

Respiratory System: Take a deep breath, and you're engaging your respiratory system. Your lungs are the body's air purification plant, extracting life-sustaining oxygen from the air and expelling waste gases like carbon dioxide.

Digestive System: Time for a meal? Your digestive system swings into action. Think of your stomach as a blender, your intestines as a nutrient extractor, and your liver as the body's chemical factory. It all works together to process food, extract nutrients, and eliminate waste.

Nervous System: Your brain and nervous system are the command centre of this remarkable machine. They control your thoughts, actions, and even the involuntary processes like your heartbeat. It's the ultimate computer, processing trillions of bits of information every second.

Endocrine System: The endocrine system, often called the body's hormonal control centre, is like a network of messengers. It regulates countless bodily functions, from growth to metabolism. Your glands produce hormones, the body's chemical signals, ensuring harmony.

Immune System: Think of your immune system as the body's defense force. It's constantly on guard, identifying and combating invaders such as viruses, bacteria, and other threats. It's your own personal superhero squad.

Reproductive System: Lastly, the reproductive system, the biological key to the continuation of our species. It's the intricate dance of hormones, organs, and cells that allows life to be passed from one generation to the next.

Picture all these systems working together in perfect harmony, an orchestration so precise it's almost beyond imagination. It's as if each cell, organ, and system understand its role in this grand symphony of life.

Understanding your body is not just about appreciating its intricate design but about becoming an active participant in its upkeep and maintenance. Knowledge of your body empowers you to make informed choices, prioritize self-care, and ultimately lead a healthier, more fulfilling life.

When you understand how your body functions, you become the master conductor of your life's symphony. Here are a few reasons why this knowledge is crucial:

Preventative Health: By recognizing how your body works, you can take proactive steps to prevent illness and maintain good health. It's easier to prevent a problem than to fix it.

Better Communication: Understanding your body allows you to communicate more effectively with healthcare professionals. You can describe your symptoms and concerns with greater accuracy, leading to more precise diagnoses and treatments.

Lifestyle Choices: Knowledge of your body helps you make informed choices about your diet, exercise, and overall lifestyle. You can tailor your habits to promote a healthier and more vibrant you.

Empowerment: With insight into your body, you take control of your well-being. You become the driver rather than a passenger in the journey of your life.

As you continue reading this book, you'll delve deeper into the intricate mechanisms that make up your body, empowering you to be your own doctor, to some extent. You'll learn how to nourish your body, exercise effectively, and recognize signs of trouble. In essence, you'll become a more informed and active participant in the incredible symphony that is your life.

Welcome to a journey of discovery, empowerment, and better health. Your body is a miraculous machine; it's time to understand it, respect it, and care for it like the treasure it is.

CHAPTER TWO

Nourishing Your Way to Wellness: The Art of
Nutrition and Diet

In our fast-paced world, where information bombards us from every
direction, it's easy to get lost in the maze of diet trends, miracle
supplements, and conflicting advice. But amidst this chaos, one
fundamental truth remains: nutrition is the cornerstone of a healthy
life. This is the story we'll unravel in this comprehensive guide to
nutrition and diet.

Basics of Nutrition

Imagine your body as a finely tuned machine. Every day, it needs a
specific blend of nutrients to run efficiently, just like your car needs
the right fuel. Understanding the basics of nutrition is the first step
to becoming your own doctor. It's the blueprint for making informed
choices about what you eat.

At its core, nutrition is about macronutrients (carbohydrates,
proteins, and fats) and micronutrients (vitamins and minerals).

These are the building blocks of your health. For example, carbohydrates provide energy, proteins repair tissues, and fats are essential for many bodily functions.

Creating a Balanced Diet

Balancing your diet is like crafting a masterpiece. It's about ensuring you get the right nutrients in the right proportions to support your overall health and well-being. Let's delve deeper into creating a balanced diet with some practical examples.

1. Fruits and Vegetables:

Fruits and vegetables are the foundation of a balanced diet. They provide essential vitamins, minerals, fibre, and antioxidants. Aim to fill half your plate with these colourful wonders.

Examples:

Berries: Blueberries, strawberries, and raspberries are rich in antioxidants and vitamin C.

Leafy Greens: Spinach, kale, and Swiss chard are packed with vitamins A, C, and K.

Citrus Fruits: Oranges, grapefruits, and lemons are bursting with vitamin C.

Cruciferous Vegetables: Broccoli, cauliflower, and Brussels sprouts are high in fibre and nutrients.

Root Vegetables: Sweet potatoes and carrots provide vitamin A and fibre.

2. Whole Grains:

Whole grains are an excellent source of complex carbohydrates, which provide sustained energy and essential nutrients.

Examples:

Oats: Rich in fibre and known for lowering cholesterol levels.

Quinoa: A complete protein source and high in fibre.

Brown Rice: Provides energy and essential minerals like magnesium.

Whole Wheat Bread: A good source of fibre and B vitamins.

Barley: High in fibre and supports heart health.

3. Lean Proteins:

Proteins are the building blocks of muscles and tissues. Opt for lean sources to reduce saturated fat intake.

Examples:

Skinless Poultry: Chicken and turkey are low in fat and rich in protein.

Fish: Fatty fish like salmon, trout, and mackerel are packed with omega-3 fatty acids.

Legumes: Beans, lentils, and chickpeas are excellent plant-based protein sources.

Tofu: A versatile source of protein for vegetarians and vegans.

Eggs: A complete protein source with essential amino acids.

4. Healthy Fats:

Healthy fats are crucial for overall health, supporting brain function, cell growth, and the absorption of certain vitamins.

Examples:

Avocado: Rich in monounsaturated fats and fibre.

Nuts and Seeds: Almonds, walnuts, chia seeds, and flaxseeds are packed with healthy fats.

Olive Oil: Extra virgin olive oil is a staple of the Mediterranean diet.

Fatty Fish: As mentioned earlier, they contain heart-healthy omega-3 fatty acids.

Coconut Oil: A source of medium-chain triglycerides (MCTs) with various potential health benefits.

5. Dairy or Dairy Alternatives:

Dairy products are a source of calcium, vitamin D, and protein. If you're lactose intolerant or choose not to consume dairy, there are alternatives available.

Examples:

Milk: Whole, low-fat, or non-fat dairy milk options.

Yogurt: Greek yogurt, regular yogurt, and dairy-free yogurt alternatives.

Cheese: Varieties like cheddar, mozzarella, and dairy-free cheese.

Almond Milk: A popular dairy milk substitute.

Soy Milk: A rich source of plant-based protein.

Remember, the magic lies in the proportions. The famous "plate method" suggests that around half your plate should be filled with fruits and vegetables, a quarter with lean proteins, and a quarter with whole grains. Healthy fats and dairy (or alternatives) should complement your meal in appropriate quantities.

Creating a balanced diet is a journey, and it's essential to enjoy a variety of foods to ensure you receive a wide range of nutrients. Additionally, portion control is key to maintaining a healthy balance. Consulting with a registered dietitian can provide personalized guidance tailored to your specific needs and preferences.

Special Diets for Specific Needs

There's no one-size-fits-all when it comes to diets. Our bodies are as unique as our fingerprints. Depending on your lifestyle, preferences, and health needs, you might want to explore specialized diets. Here are some options:

- **Mediterranean Diet:**

Description: The Mediterranean diet is a heart-healthy diet inspired by the traditional eating patterns of countries bordering the Mediterranean Sea. It's known for its emphasis on fresh fruits and vegetables, whole grains, and healthy fats, primarily from olive oil.

Key Benefits: This diet has been linked to a reduced risk of heart disease, stroke, and improved longevity.

Examples: A typical Mediterranean meal might include grilled fish, a large salad with fresh vegetables, olives, and olive oil, whole-grain bread, and a glass of red wine (in moderation).

- **Paleo Diet:**

Description: The Paleo diet is based on the idea of eating like our hunter-gatherer ancestors. It emphasizes whole foods, including lean meats, fish, fruits, vegetables, nuts, and seeds, while avoiding processed foods, grains, and dairy.

Key Benefits: Advocates of the Paleo diet claim it can lead to weight loss, improved blood sugar control, and better digestion.

Examples: A Paleo meal might consist of grilled chicken, a large serving of mixed vegetables, and a handful of nuts.

- **Vegan and Vegetarian Diets:**

Description: Veganism excludes all animal products, including meat, dairy, and eggs, while vegetarianism may allow for dairy and eggs. These diets emphasize plant-based foods and can vary in strictness.

Key Benefits: Vegan and vegetarian diets are associated with reduced risk of chronic diseases, lower cholesterol, and better weight management.

Examples: A vegan meal might include a chickpea and vegetable curry, while a vegetarian meal could be a spinach and cheese stuffed pasta.

- **Ketogenic Diet:**

Description: The ketogenic diet is a high-fat, low-carb diet that aims to put the body into a state of ketosis, where it burns fat for energy. This diet typically limits carbohydrates to 20-50 grams per day.

Key Benefits: The ketogenic diet is primarily used for weight loss, managing epilepsy, and some neurological conditions.

Examples: A ketogenic meal could consist of an avocado and bacon salad with olive oil dressing.

- **Gluten-Free Diet:**

Description: This diet eliminates foods containing gluten, a protein found in wheat, barley, and rye. It's essential for individuals with celiac disease, gluten sensitivity, or wheat allergy.

Key Benefits: A gluten-free diet prevents gastrointestinal symptoms and other health issues for those with celiac disease or gluten sensitivity.

Examples: Gluten-free meals often include foods like quinoa, rice, corn, and gluten-free pasta.

- **DASH Diet (Dietary Approaches to Stop Hypertension):**

Description: The DASH diet focuses on reducing sodium intake and includes a variety of foods, such as fruits, vegetables, lean proteins, and whole grains.

Key Benefits: It's designed to lower blood pressure and reduce the risk of heart disease.

Examples: A DASH-friendly meal might include grilled chicken, brown rice, steamed broccoli, and a side of mixed berries.

- **Low-FODMAP Diet:**

Description: This diet is designed for individuals with irritable bowel syndrome (IBS) and involves limiting foods high in fermentable carbohydrates (FODMAPs) that can trigger digestive symptoms.

Key Benefits: It can help manage IBS symptoms, including bloating and abdominal discomfort.

Examples: A low-FODMAP meal might consist of grilled chicken, white rice, and zucchini.

- **Intermittent Fasting:**

Description: Intermittent fasting is not about specific foods but focuses on when you eat. It involves cycles of eating and fasting, such as the 16/8 method (16 hours fasting, 8 hours eating).

Key Benefits: It's often used for weight management, improved insulin sensitivity, and potential longevity benefits.

Examples: During the eating window, you might have two or three balanced meals, while the fasting period involves consuming only non-caloric beverages.

Remember that the choice of a special diet should be made with careful consideration of your individual health needs and goals. It's advisable to consult with a healthcare professional or registered dietitian before making significant dietary changes, especially if you have underlying health conditions or specific dietary requirements.

CHAPTER THREE

Unlocking Your Potential: The Transformative
Power of Exercise and Physical Activity

In today's fast-paced world, where demands on our time and attention seem never-ending, it's easy to neglect one of the most essential aspects of our well-being: physical fitness. However, the benefits of exercise extend far beyond just physical health. They encompass mental, emotional, and even social well-being.

The Benefits of Exercise

Exercise is more than just a means to shed pounds or sculpt your body. It's a powerhouse for holistic well-being. Here are some of the myriad benefits that exercise brings to your life:

I.   Physical Health: Regular exercise strengthens your heart, improves circulation, and enhances your respiratory function. It can help prevent chronic diseases such as heart disease, diabetes, and obesity.

II. Mental Clarity: Exercise isn't just about building muscle; it's about building a better brain. Physical activity releases endorphins, which reduce stress and improve cognitive function. You'll think clearer and feel happier.

III. Emotional Balance: Exercise is a natural mood enhancer. It helps combat depression and anxiety by increasing the production of serotonin and norepinephrine.

IV. Weight Management: It's a powerful tool for managing your weight. A regular exercise routine helps you maintain a healthy body weight, which is crucial for overall well-being.

V. Better Sleep: Those who exercise regularly tend to enjoy more restful and restorative sleep. Say goodbye to restless nights and groggy mornings.

VI. Longevity: Exercise is a key to a longer, healthier life. Studies consistently show that active individuals live longer and enjoy a higher quality of life as they age.

Creating an Exercise Routine

Now that you're convinced of the benefits, let's dive into creating a personalized exercise routine that's sustainable and enjoyable:

➢ Set Clear Goals: Define what you want to achieve with your exercise routine. Whether it's weight loss, muscle gain, improved endurance, or better mental health, having clear goals will keep you motivated.

➢ Choose Activities You Love: Exercise doesn't have to mean monotonous gym sessions. Find activities you genuinely enjoy, whether it's dancing, hiking, swimming, or team sports. This ensures you'll look forward to staying active.

➢ Consistency is Key: A successful exercise routine relies on consistency. Set a schedule and stick to it. Start with a manageable frequency and gradually increase the intensity and duration of your workouts.

- ➤ Variety is Vital: Prevent boredom and plateaus by incorporating different types of exercises into your routine. Mix cardio, strength training, flexibility, and balance exercises.

- ➤ Track Your Progress: Keep a record of your workouts and achievements. This not only motivates you but also helps you fine-tune your routine for optimal results.

Staying Active Throughout Life

Exercise isn't just for the young; it's a lifelong commitment to well-being. Here's why staying active as you age is crucial:

- ➤ Maintaining Independence: Regular physical activity preserves your mobility, allowing you to stay independent and enjoy a high quality of life as you age.

- ➤ Reducing the Risk of Age-Related Conditions: Staying active can lower your risk of age-related conditions such as osteoporosis, arthritis, and cognitive decline.

➢ Social Engagement: Exercise can be a social activity, connecting you with like-minded individuals and fostering a sense of community.

➢ Increased Longevity: Staying active as you age isn't just about extending life, but enhancing its quality. You'll be more agile, happier, and continue to make cherished memories.

In conclusion, exercise is a gift you give to yourself. It's an investment in your physical, mental, and emotional well-being that pays extraordinary dividends. By creating a tailored exercise routine and maintaining an active lifestyle throughout life, you'll unlock your true potential and enjoy the benefits of a vibrant, fulfilling existence. Don't wait; start your journey toward a healthier, happier you today.

CHAPTER FOUR

Harmony Within: Nurturing Mental Health and Stress Management for a Balanced Life

In today's fast-paced world, the delicate balance between mental well-being and the stresses of everyday life can often seem like a tightrope walk. Our mental health is intrinsically linked to our overall well-being, and managing stress is essential for a harmonious existence. In this chapter, we'll explore the profound connection between the mind and body, uncover effective coping strategies for stress, and provide valuable insights into maintaining optimal mental health.

Mind-body Connection

The mind-body connection is a remarkable and intricate phenomenon that demonstrates how our mental and emotional well-being can significantly impact our physical health. This connection has been the subject of extensive research and study, revealing the profound ways in which our thoughts, emotions, and mental state affect our bodily functions. Let's explore this connection with a few illustrative examples:

Illustration 1: Stress and the Immune System

When you experience stress, your body's fight-or-flight response is triggered. Stress hormones like cortisol and adrenaline surge through your bloodstream, preparing your body for immediate action. While this response can be beneficial in the short term, chronic stress can weaken your immune system.

Imagine you have a demanding job that consistently causes stress. The chronic release of stress hormones can lead to reduced immune function. Over time, you might find yourself falling ill more frequently or struggling to recover from illnesses. This illustrates the direct link between your emotional state and your physical health.

Illustration 2: Emotions and Physical Pain

Emotions like sadness, anxiety, or anger can manifest physically. Consider someone dealing with chronic stress and anxiety. The persistent emotional strain might lead to muscle tension, which can cause headaches or back pain. These physical symptoms are a direct result of the emotional stress they are experiencing.

Illustration 3: The Placebo Effect

The placebo effect is a fascinating example of the mind's influence on the body. When a person believes a treatment or medication will help them, their body can exhibit real improvements, even if the treatment is inert. This shows the power of belief and positive thinking in influencing physical outcomes.

Illustration 4: Mind-Body Practices

Mind-body practices, such as yoga and meditation, demonstrate the reverse effect—how focusing on the mind can positively impact the body. Meditation, for instance, has been shown to reduce stress, lower blood pressure, and improve overall well-being. This is a clear illustration of how mental techniques can have a beneficial influence on physical health.

Illustration 5: Psychosomatic Illness

Psychosomatic illnesses are those in which psychological factors significantly contribute to physical symptoms. For example, an individual experiencing extreme anxiety might develop digestive issues like irritable bowel syndrome (IBS). The mental distress directly contributes to physical ailments.

These examples emphasize that the mind and body are not isolated entities but deeply interconnected. What happens in one can profoundly affect the other. Recognizing this connection allows us to take a more holistic approach to health and well-being, acknowledging that physical health isn't solely a matter of biology but is intricately linked to our emotions, thoughts, and mental state.

Understanding the mind-body connection underscores the importance of maintaining good mental health and managing stress effectively, as it can have a tangible impact on our overall physical health and well-being. It also highlights the significance of a holistic approach to healthcare that addresses both mental and physical aspects of wellness.

Coping with Stress

Stress can be overwhelming, but with effective coping strategies, you can navigate the storm and find calm in the chaos.

Practical strategies for coping with stress:

1. Mindfulness and Meditation:

Picture someone sitting in a quiet space, cross-legged, with their eyes closed. They are breathing deeply and slowly, fully engaged in the present moment.

Mindfulness and meditation involve focusing your attention on the here and now. This practice allows you to detach from racing thoughts and reduce the impact of stressors.

2. Physical Activity:

Show a person jogging in a park or practicing yoga. Their posture is upright, and they appear relaxed and content.

Regular physical activity, such as jogging, yoga, or even a brisk walk, releases endorphins, the body's natural mood elevators. These endorphins help reduce stress and promote a sense of well-being.

3. Breathing Techniques:

Depict a person sitting comfortably, taking a deep breath in through their nose, and exhaling slowly through their mouth. Visualize the breath traveling into their body and calming their nervous system.

Deep breathing exercises like diaphragmatic breathing or the 4-7-8 technique can activate the body's relaxation response. It lowers heart rate, reduces blood pressure, and calms stress.

4. Journaling and Self-Reflection:

Show someone with a journal, sitting in a quiet space, writing down their thoughts and emotions. There are visible pages filled with reflections and thoughts.

Journaling allows you to externalize your thoughts and feelings. It provides an opportunity to gain insights into your stressors, identify patterns, and develop coping strategies.

5. Social Support:

Visualize a person surrounded by supportive friends or family, engaged in a conversation. They are sharing their concerns and receiving comfort.

Social support is like a safety net when dealing with stress. Talking to friends, family, or a support group can offer a sense of relief, guidance, and a feeling of not being alone in your struggles.

Combining several of these strategies can offer a more comprehensive approach to managing stress, and it's a trial-and-error process to find what works best for you. Remember, the goal is not to eliminate stress entirely but to build resilience and navigate life's challenges with grace and strength.

Strategies for Maintaining Good Mental Health

Preventive measures are just as vital as stress management techniques. An array of strategies for maintaining good mental health over the long term:

Balanced Nutrition: Discover how the food you consume impacts your mental state. A well-rounded diet can provide essential nutrients that support brain health.

Adequate Sleep: Unearth the power of quality sleep in enhancing mood, cognitive function, and emotional resilience.

Setting Realistic Goals: Learn how to set achievable goals and manage expectations, reducing unnecessary stress.

Embracing Positive Thinking: Harness the transformative power of positive thinking and gratitude in your daily life.

Seeking Professional Help: Understand when it's time to reach out to mental health professionals. They can offer guidance and therapy tailored to your specific needs.

Invest in your mental health. Embrace the mind-body connection. Discover effective stress management techniques. And nurture the well-balanced, healthy life you deserve. Your path to a harmonious existence begins here

CHAPTER FIVE

Invest in Your Health: The Power of Preventive Care

In a world where the demands of daily life can sometimes feel overwhelming, our health often takes a backseat. The modern pace of life can be relentless, leaving little time to consider our well-being until a health crisis strikes. But what if I told you that there is a way to take control of your health, potentially preventing serious illnesses and ensuring a longer, healthier life? It's all about the power of preventive care.

The Importance of Preventive Health Measures

Preventive health measures are the cornerstone of a healthier, more fulfilling life. They encompass a range of practices, from lifestyle choices to routine medical check-ups, all with one goal in mind: safeguarding your well-being. The significance of these measures cannot be overstated.

A proactive approach to health means identifying potential issues before they escalate into major concerns. By investing in preventive care, you are taking charge of your health narrative and making choices that can lead to a better quality of life. Preventive care not only saves lives but also enhances the overall quality of life. It's about staying ahead of the curve and enjoying a sense of well-being that comes with knowing you've done your best to stay healthy.

Regular Check-Ups and Screenings

One of the fundamental elements of preventive care is the routine medical check-up. These appointments are not just about addressing existing health issues; they are about preventing them in the first place. Regular check-ups serve as a vital tool in early detection, enabling healthcare providers to spot potential problems before they become critical.

During these visits, your healthcare provider will perform a series of assessments, including blood pressure checks, cholesterol screenings, and physical examinations. These tests can reveal risk factors and health conditions that may not display noticeable symptoms. The earlier these issues are identified, the more effectively they can be managed, often preventing more serious health complications down the road.

Screenings are tailored to an individual's age, gender, and risk factors, with some of the most common including mammograms, Pap smears, and colonoscopies. These screenings are pivotal in the early diagnosis of conditions like breast cancer, cervical cancer, and colorectal cancer, providing a window of opportunity for effective treatment and improved outcomes.

Vaccinations and Immunizations

Vaccinations and immunizations are among the most successful public health interventions in history. They have saved countless lives and prevented numerous serious diseases. The principle behind vaccines is simple yet profound: they stimulate your immune system to recognize and fight specific pathogens, thereby preventing infection.

Childhood vaccinations are well-known and have significantly reduced the incidence of diseases such as measles, mumps, and polio. However, vaccines are not just for kids; they are crucial for adults too. Influenza, pneumonia, and shingles vaccines are recommended for adults, especially for those over 65 or with specific risk factors.

Furthermore, recent years have seen ground-breaking developments in vaccines, with COVID-19 vaccines being a remarkable example. These vaccines have proven that scientific advancements can be instrumental in protecting the global population against a novel and deadly virus. They have not only reduced the spread of the virus but also prevented severe illness and death.

By getting vaccinated, you are not only protecting yourself but also contributing to herd immunity, making it harder for diseases to spread within your community.

The Economics of Preventive Care

Preventive care isn't just a boon for your health; it can also be a smart financial choice. Preventing illnesses and catching them early through regular check-ups and screenings can lead to significant cost savings.

Treating chronic illnesses or severe health conditions often requires substantial medical expenses, hospital stays, and medications. Preventing these conditions can help you avoid the financial burden associated with severe medical interventions. Furthermore, early detection of certain diseases means that they can be managed with less invasive and less costly treatments.

Moreover, preventive care can reduce the number of missed workdays and boost overall productivity. When you're healthy, you're more likely to excel at work and enjoy a better quality of life.

In a world that's constantly in motion, our health is a precious asset that deserves our utmost attention. Preventive care is your key to ensuring a long, healthy, and fulfilling life. It's about taking charge of your health and making choices that positively impact your future.

By embracing regular check-ups, screenings, and vaccinations, you are not only safeguarding your well-being but also contributing to a healthier society. Moreover, you are making a smart financial investment that can save you from costly medical bills down the road.

So, the next time you're tempted to postpone that doctor's appointment or hesitate to get a vaccination, remember that you hold the power to shape your health and your future. Invest in your health, for a healthier you, and a brighter tomorrow. Your well-being is worth it.

CHAPTER SIX

Common Ailments and Home Remedies: Your
Ultimate Guide to Self-Care

In a world where health is paramount, we often encounter minor

ailments and discomforts that can throw a wrench into our daily

routines. These common afflictions, from the nagging sore throat to

the occasional headache, don't always require a trip to the doctor.

Instead, armed with knowledge and simple home remedies, you can

empower yourself to be your own healer. This guide explores self-

care for minor illnesses, first aid techniques, herbal remedies, and

alternative therapies that will help you stay healthy and vibrant.

Self-care for minor illnesses is an essential skill to have, as it empowers you to manage common ailments effectively. Self-care techniques for several minor illnesses:

1. The Common Cold and Flu:

Rest: Rest is crucial for recovery. It allows your body to divert energy towards healing.

Stay Hydrated: Drink plenty of water, clear broths, and herbal teas to stay hydrated. This helps thin mucus and soothes a sore throat.

Warm Salt Gargle: Gargling with warm salt water can ease throat discomfort.

Over-the-Counter Medications: Over-the-counter (OTC) cold and flu remedies can relieve symptoms such as congestion, cough, and fever. Follow the recommended dosages.

2. Sore Throat and Cough:

Hydration: As with a cold, keeping hydrated is essential.

Honey and Lemon: A mixture of honey and lemon can soothe a sore throat and suppress cough.

Throat Lozenges: Medicated throat lozenges can temporarily relieve throat discomfort.

3. Headaches and Migraines:

Hydration: Dehydration can be a headache trigger, so ensure you drink enough water.

Rest and Dark Room: Lie down in a dark, quiet room if you have a migraine. Reducing sensory input can help.

Caffeine: A small amount of caffeine can alleviate some headaches.

OTC Pain Relievers: OTC pain relievers like ibuprofen or aspirin can help relieve headache pain.

4. Upset Stomach and Indigestion:

Ginger: Ginger tea or ginger chews can ease nausea and indigestion.

Mint: Peppermint tea or peppermint oil capsules can provide relief.

Small, Frequent Meals: Eating smaller meals more often can help prevent indigestion.

Avoid Trigger Foods: Identify and avoid foods that worsen your symptoms.

5. Allergies:

Antihistamines: OTC antihistamines can help manage allergy symptoms.

Nasal Irrigation: A saline nasal rinse can clear allergens from your nasal passages.

Keep Windows Closed: Reducing exposure to outdoor allergens can help.

➢ Rest: Give your body the time it needs to heal.

➢ Maintain Good Hygiene: Wash your hands frequently to prevent the spread of illness.

➢ Isolate Yourself: If you're contagious, try to minimize contact with others to prevent the spread of illness.

➢ Seek Professional Help When Needed: If symptoms worsen, persist, or you have a high fever, it's important to consult a healthcare professional.

Remember, self-care for minor illnesses is about symptom relief and supporting your body's natural healing processes. It's not a replacement for professional medical advice, especially if you have chronic conditions or severe symptoms. Always consult a healthcare provider when in doubt or if symptoms are severe or long-lasting.

Accidents and minor injuries can happen anytime, anywhere. Being well-prepared and knowing first aid techniques can make all the difference in an emergency. Some essential first aid techniques and how to perform them:

1. **Cuts and Wounds:**

   a. **Cleaning:**

   ➤ Start by washing your hands thoroughly to avoid introducing bacteria.

   ➤ Use mild soap and clean, lukewarm water to gently cleanse the wound.

   ➤ Avoid using hydrogen peroxide or alcohol, as they can damage tissue.

   ➤ Pat the area dry with a clean cloth or sterile gauze.

   b. **Disinfection**:

   ➤ Apply an antiseptic solution, like hydrogen peroxide, iodine, or an over-the-counter wound disinfectant.

➤ Use a sterile cotton ball or gauze to apply the antiseptic to the wound.

➤ Ensure the disinfectant doesn't come into direct contact with the surrounding healthy skin.

c. Bandaging:

➤ Use sterile gauze or adhesive bandages to cover the wound.

➤ Apply gentle pressure to control bleeding.

➤ If the wound is deep or gaping, it may require stitches, and you should seek medical attention.

2. Burns and Scalds:

a. Cool the Burn:

➤ Hold the affected area under cold, running water for about 10-20 minutes.

➤ If water is not available, use a cold, damp cloth to cool the burn.

b. Protect the Burn:

➢ Cover the burn with a clean, non-stick bandage or plastic wrap to prevent infection.

➢ Avoid using adhesive bandages directly on burns.

c. Pain Relief:

➢ Over-the-counter pain relievers like ibuprofen can help alleviate pain and reduce inflammation.

➢ Do not use ice, as it can damage the burned tissue.

3. Sprains and Strains:

a. Rest:

➢ Avoid putting weight on the injured area.

➢ Use crutches or a brace if necessary, to stabilize the injury.

b. Ice:

Apply an ice pack wrapped in a thin cloth for 15-20 minutes every 1-2 hours during the first 48 hours to reduce swelling and pain.

c. Compression:

➢ Use an elastic bandage to gently compress the injured area to reduce swelling.

➢ Make sure it's snug but not too tight, as it can impede circulation.

    d. **Elevation**:

Elevate the injured limb above heart level when possible to reduce swelling.

4. **Insect Bites and Stings:**

    a. **Remove the Stinger:**

➢ For bee stings, gently scrape the stinger out with a flat-edged object. Do not pinch or use tweezers, as this may inject more venom.

➢ For tick bites, use fine-tipped tweezers to grasp the tick as close to the skin's surface as possible and pull upward with steady, even pressure.

    b. **Clean the Area:**

➢ Wash the bite or sting site with soap and water.

➢ Apply an antiseptic to prevent infection.

c. Reduce Swelling:

➢ Apply a cold compress to the bite or sting site for 10-15 minutes to reduce pain and swelling.

➢ Over-the-counter antihistamines or pain relievers may also help.

These are some fundamental first aid techniques for common injuries. Always seek professional medical attention if the injury is severe, the person's condition worsens, or if you're uncertain about how to handle the situation. Proper first aid knowledge and actions can make a significant difference in recovery and the prevention of complications.

Nature has provided us with a treasure trove of remedies that have been used for centuries. Herbal remedies and alternative therapies offer gentle yet effective solutions to many common ailments.

Aloe vera: A versatile healing plant for skin irritations and minor burns.

Ginger: Nature's remedy for nausea, indigestion, and inflammation.

Lavender: A soothing herb for stress, anxiety, and sleep troubles.

Eucalyptus: A respiratory relief for congestion and cold symptoms.

Arnica: A natural anti-inflammatory for muscle aches and bruises.

But, it's essential to approach these remedies with care and caution.

Empower Yourself with Knowledge

This guide empowers you to take control of your health. By understanding common ailments and having practical remedies at your fingertips, you can speed up your recovery, relieve discomfort, and regain your vitality. Knowledge is your best tool for self-care.

Don't let minor ailments slow you down. With the wisdom in this guide, you'll have the confidence to tackle common illnesses head-on, provide first aid in emergencies, and explore the world of natural healing through herbs and alternative therapies. Your health is in your hands, and this guide will equip you with the knowledge to make the best decisions for your well-being.

In an age where self-care is becoming increasingly important, "Common Ailments and Home Remedies: Your Ultimate Guide to Self-Care" is your trusted companion on the journey to a healthier, happier you. Say goodbye to minor ailments, and embrace a life of vitality and well-being. Get your copy today and become your own best healer. Your health is worth it.

CHAPTER SEVEN

Chronic Disease Management: Taking Control of Your Health

Chronic conditions are relentless adversaries, from diabetes to heart disease, asthma to arthritis. But the power of understanding and proactively managing them can change the game. By equipping yourself with knowledge, you can shift from a passive observer to an empowered participant in your healthcare journey.

One of the cornerstones of chronic disease management is regular medical check-ups. These appointments serve as a compass guiding your health journey. They help in early detection, accurate diagnosis, and tracking the progress of your condition. The insights gained from these appointments are invaluable.

But it doesn't stop there. Medication management plays a pivotal role in chronic disease management. Prescription drugs can control symptoms, prevent complications, and slow disease progression. However, understanding your medications, their side effects, and adhering to your doctor's recommendations is crucial. Your medication regimen is your partner in this journey, working alongside you to keep your condition in check.

Medication Management: Your Pillars of Support

Proper medication management can be life-changing. The first step is to engage in an open and honest dialogue with your healthcare provider. Share your concerns, questions, and any side effects you might be experiencing. Collaboration is key, as your healthcare team can make necessary adjustments to your medication plan based on your unique needs.

In today's digital age, medication management apps and reminders have become valuable allies in the fight against chronic conditions. They help you stay organized and ensure you never miss a dose. These tools allow you to track your progress, providing insights that can be discussed with your healthcare provider during your visits.

Adherence is paramount when it comes to medication management. Skipping doses or discontinuing medication can have severe consequences. Remember, your medications are specifically prescribed to help manage your condition and improve your quality of life. Be consistent, ask questions, and never hesitate to seek clarification from your healthcare team.

Lifestyle Changes for Chronic Conditions: Your Path to a Brighter Tomorrow

Lifestyle changes are the unsung heroes in the realm of chronic disease management. They complement medication, reinforce your health, and empower you to lead a fuller life.

Nutrition: Your dietary choices can significantly impact your chronic condition. Consult with a nutritionist or dietitian to create a customized meal plan. Focus on a balanced diet rich in whole foods, fruits, vegetables, and lean proteins. Minimize your intake of processed and sugary foods.

Physical Activity: Regular exercise can improve your condition by increasing your strength, endurance, and overall well-being. Consult your healthcare provider to develop an exercise plan tailored to your abilities and limitations.

Stress Management: Chronic conditions often bring stress. Learning stress management techniques, such as meditation, yoga, or deep breathing exercises, can help reduce stress and improve your overall health.

Sleep: Quality sleep is essential for the body's healing and recovery. Maintain a regular sleep schedule and create a comfortable sleeping environment.

Support System: Chronic conditions can be emotionally challenging. Building a strong support network of friends, family, or support groups can help you navigate the emotional aspects of managing your condition.

Remember that these lifestyle changes are a continuous journey, and it's okay to take small steps. Progress may be slow, but every positive choice you make is a victory on your path to wellness.

Chronic disease management, medication management, and lifestyle changes are the three pillars that can empower you to lead a fulfilling life. By understanding your condition, collaborating with healthcare providers, and making proactive lifestyle changes, you're taking a significant step towards a brighter and healthier future.

CHAPTER EIGHT

Empowering Yourself through Self-Diagnosis and Symptom Management

In an age of information accessibility, the ability to identify symptoms and manage one's health has never been more crucial. This article explores the essential aspects of self-diagnosis and symptom management, empowering individuals to take an active role in their well-being. We'll delve into the art of identifying symptoms, the use of online health resources, and the critical decision of when to seek professional help.

Identifying Symptoms

Understanding and accurately recognizing symptoms is a fundamental step in self-diagnosis and symptom management. Here's a more detailed exploration:

1. The Body's Language:

Our bodies are complex systems that have evolved to communicate distress or dysfunction through a language of symptoms. Symptoms are essentially signals that something is amiss within the body. They can manifest in various ways, including but not limited to:

➢ Pain: Pain can occur in various forms – sharp, dull, throbbing, or aching. It may be localized or widespread, and its intensity can vary.

➢ Discomfort: Discomfort encompasses feelings of unease, irritation, or inconvenience. This can be physical discomfort, like an upset stomach, or emotional discomfort, like anxiety.

➤ Changes in Appearance: Some symptoms are visible, such as rashes, discoloration, swelling, or changes in skin texture. Paying attention to such changes is crucial.

➤ Altered Bodily Functions: Changes in bodily functions, such as digestion, urination, or bowel movements, can be significant symptoms. These changes can include constipation, diarrhoea, blood in urine, or changes in menstrual patterns.

2. Know Your Baseline:

To effectively identify symptoms, it's important to have a clear understanding of what's normal for your body. This means being aware of your baseline health status. Everyone's body is unique, and what's normal for one person might not be normal for another. Knowing your baseline allows you to recognize deviations from it. Here are some steps to establish your baseline:

➤ Regular Check-Ups: Periodic check-ups with a healthcare provider can help establish your baseline health status. They can provide you with important metrics like blood pressure, cholesterol levels, and body mass index (BMI).

➤ Self-Reflection: Take time to reflect on your typical physical and mental state. Are you usually energetic, or do you tend to feel fatigued? What's your typical body temperature? How does your skin normally look and feel?

3. Track Your Symptoms:

Maintaining a symptom journal can be an invaluable tool in symptom management. Recording your symptoms allows for a more systematic approach to self-diagnosis. Here's how to create and use a symptom journal:

➤ Record Details: Note the date, time, and duration of each symptom. Include the location of the symptom and its intensity. Describe what you're experiencing in as much detail as possible.

➢ Include Triggers: Identify any potential triggers or patterns. For instance, you might notice that your headaches tend to occur after consuming certain foods or when you're stressed.

➢ Monitor Changes: Over time, review your symptom journal to track any changes or trends. Are symptoms improving, worsening, or staying the same? This information can be invaluable when discussing your condition with a healthcare professional.

By understanding the body's language, knowing your baseline, and systematically tracking your symptoms, you'll be better equipped to identify and manage health-related issues. It's important to remember that while self-diagnosis is a valuable skill, it should be complemented by professional medical advice, especially in the case of severe or chronic conditions.

Online health resources play a crucial role in empowering individuals to make informed decisions about their health. These resources are readily available on the internet and provide a wealth of information related to various health conditions, symptoms, treatments, and preventive measures. Different aspects of online health resources:

Information Accessibility:

The internet has democratized access to health information. Online health resources encompass websites, databases, articles, videos, and forums that cover a wide range of health-related topics. This accessibility allows people to learn about different health conditions, symptoms, and treatments from the comfort of their homes.

Reputable Sources:

It's crucial to rely on reputable sources for accurate and trustworthy health information. Government health agencies, well-established medical institutions, and respected medical websites like Mayo Clinic, WebMD, and the Centres for Disease Control and Prevention (CDC) are examples of such sources. These organizations are known for their commitment to evidence-based information.

Symptom Checkers:

Symptom checkers are interactive tools available on various health websites and apps. Users can input their symptoms, and the tool provides a list of potential conditions that may be associated with those symptoms. While symptom checkers can be helpful for narrowing down possibilities, they should not replace professional medical advice, diagnosis, or treatment.

Understanding Medical Terminology:

Online health resources often use medical terminology and jargon. It's beneficial for individuals to familiarize themselves with common medical terms, as this enhances their ability to comprehend and interpret the information they find. Online medical dictionaries and glossaries can be valuable in this regard.

Researching Specific Conditions:

Online resources enable individuals to research specific health conditions. They can learn about the causes, symptoms, risk factors, and available treatments for a particular ailment. This knowledge can help individuals engage in more informed discussions with healthcare providers.

Treatment Options and Guidelines:

Online health resources often provide information about available treatment options for various conditions. This includes details about medications, therapies, surgeries, and lifestyle changes that may be recommended. Additionally, individuals can find guidelines for managing chronic conditions and preventive measures.

Preventive Health and Wellness:

These resources are not limited to diagnosing and treating illnesses. Many of them also offer guidance on maintaining overall health and wellness. This includes articles on nutrition, exercise, stress management, and preventive healthcare measures, such as vaccinations and screenings.

Online Support Communities:

Online health resources can connect individuals with support communities and forums where they can interact with people who share similar health concerns. These communities provide a platform for sharing experiences, advice, and emotional support, contributing to a sense of belonging and understanding.

Health Apps and Wearables:

Mobile applications and wearable devices are increasingly used as health resources. These tools can track various health metrics, such as heart rate, sleep patterns, and physical activity. They offer insights into an individual's health status and can encourage healthier lifestyle choices.

It's important to note that while online health resources are valuable, they should complement, not replace, professional medical advice. Self-diagnosis and self-treatment based solely on online information can be risky, especially for complex or serious medical conditions. It's always advisable to consult a healthcare provider for a proper diagnosis and personalized medical guidance.

Recognizing the right time to consult a healthcare professional is essential for timely diagnosis and effective treatment. Here are key factors to consider:

1. Trust Your Gut Instinct:

Your intuition is a valuable tool. If you have a strong feeling that something is wrong or that your symptoms are not normal, trust your instincts. While not a definitive indicator, gut feelings can be an important prompt to seek professional advice.

2. Symptoms of Urgency:

Certain symptoms demand immediate medical attention, and delaying could have severe consequences. These include:

➢ Chest Pain: Chest pain, especially if it radiates to the arm, neck, or jaw, could be a sign of a heart attack.

➢ Severe Bleeding: Uncontrolled or heavy bleeding requires urgent care.

85

- ➤ Loss of Consciousness: Fainting or losing consciousness should not be ignored.

- ➤ Signs of a Stroke: Sudden numbness or weakness in the face, arm, or leg, especially if it's one-sided, along with confusion, trouble speaking, or severe headache, may indicate a stroke.

In these cases, call 911 or go to the nearest emergency room immediately. Time can be a critical factor in saving lives.

3. Duration and Progression:

Pay attention to how your symptoms evolve over time. Persistent or worsening symptoms should raise concern:

- ➤ Persistent Symptoms: If a symptom lingers for an extended period, it may be a sign of an underlying condition that requires investigation.

- ➤ Interference with Daily Life: If your symptoms hinder your ability to perform daily tasks or affect your quality of life, it's time to consult a healthcare professional.

4. Chronic Conditions:

If you suspect you have a chronic condition based on recurring or long-term symptoms, it's essential to consult a healthcare provider for a proper diagnosis and management plan. Chronic conditions may include diabetes, hypertension, asthma, or autoimmune disorders. Timely management can help improve your long-term health.

5. Avoid Self-Diagnosing Serious Conditions:

While self-diagnosis is a valuable starting point, it should not be used for serious or life-threatening conditions. Attempting to self-diagnose complex or severe ailments can lead to delayed treatment and potential harm.

6. Unexplained Weight Loss:

If you're experiencing unexplained and unintentional weight loss, it can be a sign of an underlying health issue. Consult a healthcare professional to rule out serious conditions like cancer, thyroid disorders, or digestive problems.

7. Changes in Cognitive Function:

Any noticeable changes in cognitive function, such as memory loss, confusion, or disorientation, should be taken seriously. These could be indicative of neurological issues like Alzheimer's disease or other cognitive disorders.

8. Abnormal Laboratory Results:

If you have access to your medical test results and notice abnormal values, it's important to discuss these with a healthcare provider. They can provide insight into potential underlying conditions that may require further evaluation and treatment.

Knowing when to seek professional help is crucial for maintaining your health. While self-awareness and self-diagnosis are valuable tools, they should complement, not replace, the expertise of healthcare professionals. The decision to seek medical assistance should be based on a combination of factors, including your intuition, the nature and urgency of your symptoms, and a commitment to proactive healthcare. Always prioritize your well-being and consult a healthcare provider when in doubt.

CHAPTER NINE

The Healing Power of Nature: Herbal Medicine and Alternative Therapies

In a world dominated by modern medicine, the age-old wisdom of herbal remedies and alternative therapies often takes a back seat. However, these natural and holistic approaches to healing have been practiced for centuries and continue to offer valuable insights into maintaining health and well-being.

Herbal Remedies: The Gifts of the Earth

Herbal remedies are a treasure trove of nature's healing potential. These remedies are derived from plants, and their use dates back to ancient civilizations. They offer an array of benefits, from relieving common ailments to promoting overall wellness. Here are some key points to consider:

> ➤ Ancient Wisdom: Herbal remedies have been used across cultures for thousands of years. From Traditional Chinese

Medicine to Ayurveda in India, these ancient systems recognize the therapeutic value of plants.

➢ Balancing the Body: Herbal remedies often work by bringing balance to the body. They can address the root causes of illnesses and provide long-term solutions.

➢ Holistic Approach: Herbal medicine considers the body as a whole, focusing on not just symptoms but the overall well-being of the individual.

➢ Common Herbal Remedies: Explore the world of herbal remedies, from chamomile for relaxation to ginger for digestion and echinacea for immune support.

Acupuncture and Ayurveda: Ancient Wisdom in Modern Times

Acupuncture and Ayurveda are two well-known alternative therapies that have gained recognition and respect in the Western world. These ancient practices offer unique perspectives on healing:

Acupuncture: Originating from Traditional Chinese Medicine, acupuncture involves the insertion of fine needles into specific points on the body to stimulate energy flow. It's used for a wide range of conditions, from pain management to stress relief.

Ayurveda: Ayurveda, hailing from India, is a holistic system that focuses on individual constitution and balance. It combines diet, lifestyle, and herbal treatments to promote well-being and treat a variety of conditions.

Integrative Medicine: The integration of these alternative therapies with conventional medicine is becoming more common. This approach recognizes the value of combining the best of both worlds to provide comprehensive care.

Integrating Alternative and Conventional Medicine: A New Paradigm

The integration of alternative and conventional medicine represents a paradigm shift in healthcare. Here's why it's gaining traction and how it can benefit patients:

➢ Comprehensive Care: Integrative medicine considers the whole person, addressing physical, emotional, and spiritual well-being. This approach can lead to more effective and personalized treatment plans.

➤ Patient-Centered: Patients are increasingly seeking treatments that align with their values and preferences. Integrative medicine allows patients to make choices that resonate with their beliefs and experiences.

➤ Prevention and Wellness: Integrating alternative therapies can place a greater emphasis on prevention and overall wellness, rather than just symptom management.

➤ Scientific Validation: The effectiveness of many alternative therapies is being studied rigorously, leading to scientific validation and broader acceptance in the medical community.

➤ Collaboration: Integrative medicine encourages collaboration between healthcare providers, fostering a more holistic and coordinated approach to patient care.

A Balancing Act: Choosing the Right Path

While the potential benefits of herbal medicine and alternative therapies are vast, it's essential to approach them with awareness and discernment:

➢ Consult a Professional: Always consult a qualified healthcare provider before embarking on any herbal or alternative treatment. They can offer guidance and ensure safety.

➢ Personalization: What works for one person may not work for another. Personalization and individualization are crucial when exploring alternative therapies.

➢ Research and Education: Stay informed about the therapies you're interested in. Understand their mechanisms, potential side effects, and any contraindications.

➢ Respect Tradition: Acknowledge the cultural and historical significance of these therapies. They are the result of centuries of wisdom and experience.

In a world where health and well-being are of paramount importance, the wisdom of herbal medicine and alternative therapies offers valuable insights. Whether seeking relief from a common ailment or striving for holistic well-being, these approaches empower individuals to take an active role in their health journey. The integration of these ancient practices with modern medicine presents a promising future where healing is truly comprehensive and patient-centered.

CHAPTER TEN

Building a Holistic Health Plan: A Path to Wellness and Vitality

In our fast-paced world, where daily demands often leave us feeling overwhelmed and stressed, it's easy to neglect our most precious asset—our health. We frequently find ourselves caught up in the whirlwind of life, leaving little time for self-care and well-being. However, taking a proactive approach to our health is essential for not only extending our lifespan but also enhancing our quality of life. This is where the concept of a Holistic Health Plan comes into play.

Personalized Health Goals: Crafting Your Wellness Blueprint

The journey to better health begins with setting personalized health goals. No two individuals are the same, and the path to well-being can vary greatly from one person to another. Personalized health goals help us understand what we want to achieve in terms of our health and well-being. They serve as our guiding star, providing direction and motivation for the journey ahead.

Your personalized health goals should be specific, measurable, achievable, relevant, and time-bound, often referred to as SMART goals. For instance, if you want to improve your physical fitness, a SMART goal might be: "I will walk for 30 minutes five days a week for the next three months." This goal is specific (walking), measurable (30 minutes), achievable (five days a week), relevant to your health, and time-bound (three months).

As you set your goals, consider various aspects of your health, including physical fitness, mental well-being, nutrition, and stress management. By addressing these different facets of health, you create a comprehensive picture of what well-being means to you.

Once you've established your personalized health goals, the next step is to develop a wellness routine that aligns with these objectives. This routine should encompass a wide range of activities and practices that cater to your holistic well-being. Here's a breakdown of what it could entail:

Physical Activity: Regular exercise is fundamental to a holistic health plan. It not only helps maintain a healthy weight but also improves cardiovascular health, reduces the risk of chronic diseases, and boosts mental well-being. Find an activity you enjoy, whether it's walking, running, yoga, or dancing, and incorporate it into your daily routine.

> Nutrition: What you put into your body has a profound impact on your health. A well-balanced diet, rich in fruits, vegetables, lean proteins, and whole grains, is key to

maintaining good health. Consider consulting with a nutritionist to create a meal plan that aligns with your goals.

➤ Mental Health: Caring for your mental well-being is just as important as physical health. Incorporate relaxation techniques, mindfulness, and stress management practices into your daily routine. Make time for hobbies and activities that bring you joy and reduce stress.

➤ Sleep: Adequate sleep is crucial for overall health. Develop healthy sleep habits, including a consistent sleep schedule and creating a comfortable sleep environment.

➤ Social Connections: Human beings are inherently social creatures. Nurturing positive relationships and spending time with loved ones can greatly impact your mental and emotional health.

➤ Regular Check-Ups: Don't forget the importance of regular medical check-ups to catch and address health issues early.

➢ Hydration: Proper hydration is often overlooked but is essential for optimal bodily function. Ensure you drink enough water throughout the day.

Staying Informed and Adapting: The Dynamic Nature of Health

A holistic health plan is not set in stone. It's a dynamic blueprint for well-being that needs regular evaluation and adjustment. Staying informed about the latest developments in health and wellness is crucial. Attend seminars, read books, and follow credible health websites to stay updated.

Incorporate feedback loops into your health routine. Regularly assess your progress towards your goals and be willing to adapt. If you notice that a particular aspect of your wellness routine isn't yielding the desired results, be open to modifying it. Health is not a one-size-fits-all concept, and your plan should evolve as your needs change.

Remember that setbacks and challenges are a natural part of any health journey. When faced with obstacles, don't be discouraged. Instead, view them as opportunities for growth and learning. Be compassionate with yourself and stay committed to your health goals.

In conclusion, crafting a Holistic Health Plan involves setting personalized health goals, developing a wellness routine, and staying informed and adaptable. By taking a proactive approach to your health, you can enhance your well-being and vitality, ensuring that you have the energy and resilience to fully embrace life's adventures. Your health is your most valuable asset—invest in it wisely.

CHAPTER ELEVEN

Medical Emergencies and When to Seek Professional Help.

Recognizing True Emergencies

Medical emergencies can happen at any time and can be a frightening experience. The ability to recognize a true medical emergency is crucial for your safety and the safety of those around you. Here are some key points to consider when determining if a situation constitutes a true emergency:

➤ Life-Threatening Situations: A true medical emergency often involves a life-threatening condition. If someone is experiencing severe chest pain, uncontrolled bleeding, loss of consciousness, difficulty breathing, or severe allergic reactions, these are typically red flags.

➤ Sudden and Severe Symptoms: If the symptoms come on suddenly and are severe, it's a strong indicator of an emergency. For instance, sudden weakness on one side of the body could be a sign of a stroke.

➢ Changes in Consciousness: Altered consciousness, such as confusion, disorientation, or an inability to wake someone up, is a cause for concern.

➢ Trauma: Any major injury, like a severe fall, car accident, or deep lacerations, should be considered an emergency.

➢ Severe Allergic Reactions: Symptoms like difficulty breathing, swelling of the face or throat, or severe rashes could be a sign of a severe allergic reaction, requiring immediate medical attention.

➢ Uncontrolled Bleeding: Profuse bleeding that doesn't stop with direct pressure may require emergency intervention.

Calling 911 is the fastest and most direct way to get help during a medical emergency. Here's when you should call 911:

➢ Life-Threatening Situations: If the situation is life-threatening, dial 911 immediately. Don't hesitate, as seconds can make a significant difference in these cases.

➢ Loss of Consciousness: If someone loses consciousness and doesn't wake up, this is an emergency. Inform the 911 operator of any other symptoms or details you know.

➢ Severe Chest Pain: Chest pain that lasts for more than a few minutes, especially if it radiates to the arm, jaw, or neck, could indicate a heart attack. Call 911.

➢ Severe Breathing Difficulties: If someone is struggling to breathe or turns blue, call for help.

➢ Severe Allergic Reactions: For severe allergic reactions with symptoms like difficulty breathing or swelling, dial 911.

➤ Severe Injuries: In cases of major trauma or injuries that involve broken bones, severe bleeding, or head injuries, call for an ambulance.

Preparing for Medical Appointments

While not all health-related situations are immediate emergencies, preparing for medical appointments is essential for effective care and diagnosis. Here's how to get the most out of your medical appointments:

➤ Create a Medical History: Document your medical history, including current and past illnesses, surgeries, allergies, and a list of your current medications. This information is vital for your healthcare provider to make informed decisions.

➤ List Your Concerns: Before your appointment, write down any questions or concerns you have. This will help you remember to discuss them with your doctor.

➤ Bring Relevant Information: If you have test results, images, or reports from previous medical visits, bring them to your appointment. They can provide valuable context for your healthcare provider.

➢ Follow Medication Instructions: If you're taking medication, ensure you're following the prescribed instructions and dosage. Be prepared to discuss any side effects or concerns.

➢ Know Your Family History: Understand your family's medical history as some conditions have a genetic component. This information can be crucial in assessing your risk factors.

➢ Ask for Clarification: Don't hesitate to ask your healthcare provider to clarify any medical jargon or instructions. Understanding your condition and treatment plan is essential.

In summary, recognizing a true medical emergency and knowing when to call 911 is a matter of life and death. On the other hand, effective preparation for medical appointments empowers you to take charge of your health and ensures that you receive the best care possible.

CHAPTER TWELVE

The Future of Self-Care and Health Tech

In an era where technology is advancing at an unprecedented pace, the healthcare industry is experiencing a transformation like never before. The intersection of self-care and health technology is not only changing the way individuals manage their well-being but also reshaping the entire healthcare landscape. In this article, we delve into three critical aspects of this exciting evolution: Telemedicine and Health Apps, the Role of Artificial Intelligence (AI) in Healthcare, and the ever-evolving landscape of self-care.

Telemedicine and Health Apps

Telemedicine, often referred to as "telehealth," is revolutionizing the way individuals access healthcare services. With the widespread availability of high-speed internet and the ubiquity of smartphones, telemedicine has gained significant traction. Patients can now consult with healthcare professionals remotely, saving time and eliminating geographical barriers.

Health apps play a pivotal role in this telemedicine revolution. These apps come in various forms, from symptom checkers and medication trackers to remote monitoring tools for chronic conditions. They empower individuals to actively engage in their healthcare journey. For instance, individuals with diabetes can use apps to monitor their blood sugar levels and receive real-time feedback. Mental health apps provide resources for managing stress, anxiety, and depression, promoting overall well-being.

The convenience of telemedicine and health apps is particularly evident in rural or underserved areas where access to healthcare facilities is limited. Telemedicine bridges this gap, ensuring that everyone, regardless of their location, can receive medical guidance and support. Moreover, it offers a lifeline during public health crises, as demonstrated during the COVID-19 pandemic when telehealth usage skyrocketed, enabling safe medical consultations and reducing the strain on hospitals.

Artificial Intelligence (AI) is at the forefront of healthcare innovation. AI has the potential to transform diagnostics, treatment planning, and patient care. Machine learning algorithms can analyse vast datasets more quickly and accurately than human experts. This capability enhances medical imaging, aiding radiologists in the detection of diseases like cancer and enabling early intervention.

AI-powered chatbots and virtual assistants are becoming commonplace in healthcare. They can provide personalized health advice, schedule appointments, and answer medical queries. AI's natural language processing capabilities make it easier for patients to access information and support, ultimately contributing to informed decision-making regarding self-care.

Moreover, AI-driven predictive analytics are changing the way healthcare providers approach patient care. These algorithms can identify individuals at risk of specific health conditions, allowing for proactive interventions. For example, AI can help predict heart

disease in a patient based on their medical history, lifestyle, and genetic factors, enabling preventive measures and customized treatment plans.

The Evolving Landscape of Self-Care

Self-care is no longer limited to occasional spa days and healthy eating habits. It now involves a comprehensive approach to personal health management. Individuals have access to an array of wearable devices, health monitoring tools, and online resources to track and improve their well-being continuously.

The growing focus on holistic health emphasizes the importance of mental health and emotional well-being. Mindfulness and meditation apps are empowering individuals to manage stress, anxiety, and sleep disorders. These apps guide users through relaxation techniques and offer a tranquil escape from the demands of modern life.

Self-care also extends to lifestyle choices. Wearable fitness trackers, such as smartwatches, monitor physical activity, sleep patterns, and heart rate. They provide real-time feedback to encourage users to stay active and make healthier choices. Dietary and nutrition apps assist individuals in maintaining a balanced diet, enabling them to set dietary goals, track calorie intake, and receive personalized meal plans.

The future of self-care is intertwined with personalization. Advances in technology allow for tailored approaches to health management. From genetic testing that reveals individual health predispositions to AI algorithms that recommend fitness regimens based on personal goals, self-care is becoming increasingly bespoke.

In conclusion, the future of self-care and health tech is a promising one. Telemedicine and health apps are making healthcare more accessible and convenient. AI is enhancing diagnosis, treatment, and predictive analytics, ultimately leading to better patient outcomes. The evolving landscape of self-care emphasizes holistic well-being and personalization. As these trends continue to evolve, individuals have more tools and resources at their disposal to take charge of their health and well-being, ensuring a healthier and more informed future for all.

CONCLUSION

In the concluding chapter of this book, we arrive at a pivotal moment in your journey toward becoming your own doctor. It's not just about acquiring knowledge; it's about embracing your role as a health advocate in your own life.

Empowering Yourself as a Health Advocate

Your health is a precious asset, and the power to protect and enhance it lies within you. As you've delved into the pages of this guide, you've gained insight into the intricate workings of your body, learned to make better choices in nutrition and fitness, and explored strategies to safeguard your mental well-being. Now, it's time to acknowledge the role you play in your own healthcare.

Becoming a health advocate means taking control of your health decisions, being proactive in seeking information, and being a strong, informed voice in your interactions with healthcare professionals. You have the right to ask questions, seek second opinions, and actively participate in the decision-making process when it comes to your well-being. Your journey as a health advocate doesn't replace the need for medical expertise but rather complements it, ensuring that you receive the best care possible.

Striking a Balance Between Self-Care and Professional Care

In our exploration of self-care, we've uncovered the numerous ways you can actively nurture your health, from maintaining a balanced diet to managing stress and identifying minor ailments. However, it's crucial to recognize the limits of self-care. There will be times when professional medical guidance is not just advisable but essential.

Striking a balance means knowing when to rely on your self-care skills and when to turn to healthcare professionals. It involves understanding the warning signs of serious illness, recognizing the value of regular check-ups, and realizing that your health isn't solely your responsibility; it's a partnership between you and your healthcare team.

By embracing this balance, you ensure that you receive timely, expert care when needed, while also promoting your long-term well-being through preventive self-care practices. It's the sweet spot where self-empowerment and professional expertise unite to provide you with the best possible health outcomes.

As you embark on your journey as your own doctor, remember that it's a lifelong pursuit. Your knowledge will grow, and your ability to advocate for your health will strengthen. Embrace this power, honour the importance of collaboration, and continue striving for the optimal balance between self-care and professional care. Your health is your most valuable possession, and you have the tools to protect and nurture it like no one else can.

www.ingramcontent.com/pod-product-compliance
Lightning Source LLC
Chambersburg PA
CBHW062329290526
45794CB00005B/1954